Healthy, Happy Aging:

An Essential Guide to Anti-aging

By

Marie J. Garcia

TABLE OF CONTENT

Introduction

Healthy, Happy Aging is a book that provides readers with a revolutionary guide to unlocking the secret to a healthier, happier life as they age. It explores the science of aging, discussing how the body changes and how we can adjust our lifestyle to accommodate those changes. It emphasizes the importance of exercise and nutrition, skincare, as well as the psychological aspects of aging, such as stress management, maintaining relationships, and finding joy in life. It also includes advice on dealing with changes in mobility, addressing chronic conditions, and navigating the healthcare system. By learning from experts in this field, readers can gain a better understanding of the aging process and the steps they can take to enjoy their later year.

CHAPTER 1

Aging

Aging comes with a variety of physical and emotional challenges. Many of these challenges can be addressed through lifestyle changes, such as exercising regularly and eating a nutritious diet, or through medical interventions. Some of the most common challenges associated with aging include:

1. Memory Loss: As we age, our brains tend to lose their ability to recall information quickly and accurately. Memory loss can be caused by a variety of factors, including age-related changes in the brain, medications, and health conditions such as Alzheimer's disease.

2. Mobility Issues: As we age, our bodies become less flexible and may experience joint pain and muscle weakness. These physical changes can make it difficult to move around and perform everyday tasks.

3. Social Isolation: As we age, our social circles may shrink and our opportunities to socialize may become more limited.

4. Chronic Health Conditions: As we age, our bodies become more vulnerable to chronic health conditions such as arthritis, diabetes, heart disease, and stroke.

5. Mental Health Conditions: Mental health conditions, such as depression and anxiety, can be more common in older adults.

6. Financial Concerns: Financial concerns can become more pressing as we age and as our income may decrease.

7. End-of-Life Planning: Thinking about and planning for the end of life can be difficult. However, it is important to have conversations about end-of-life wishes with family and friends.

Why is a Positive Mindset Important?

Having a positive mindset is important at any age, but it is especially important as we age. A positive attitude can help us remain optimistic and cope with the physical and mental changes that come with aging. It can also help us stay engaged in life, enjoy our relationships and activities, and maintain a sense of purpose and fulfilment.

Healthy, Happy Aging

A positive mindset can help us stay healthy by reducing stress and anxiety, improving our immune system, and promoting better sleep. It can also help us manage chronic conditions such as heart disease, diabetes, and arthritis. A positive attitude can also help us stay socially active, build meaningful relationships, and stay engaged in our community.

A positive attitude can also help us maintain our independence. It can help us stay open to new experiences and adapt to life's changes. It can also help us focus on the good things in life and make the most of our time.

Having a positive attitude can also help us maintain our mental well-being. Studies have shown that positive thinking can help reduce depression, improve self-esteem, and increase resilience. It can also help us stay motivated and take on new challenges.

In short, having a positive mindset is essential for living a healthy and fulfilling life into old age. It can help us manage physical and mental changes, stay socially active, maintain our independence, and maintain our mental well-being.

Mindful Strategies to develop a Positive Mindset

1. Practice gratitude: Take time each day to think about the things you are grateful for. Reflect on your accomplishments, relationships, and experiences that bring you joy.

2. Focus on the present moment: Don't dwell on the past or worry about the future. Instead, take time to appreciate the present moment and be mindful of any thoughts or emotions that arise.

3. Engage in Meaningful Activities: Find activities that bring you joy and purpose. This could include volunteering, learning a new skill, or connecting with family and friends.

4. Take Care of Your Health: Maintaining a healthy lifestyle is essential for your mental and physical well-being.

5. Connect with Nature: Connecting with nature is a great way to reduce stress and boost your mood. Go for a walk in the park, or enjoy some gardening or bird watching.

6. Practice Mindfulness and Meditation: Mindfulness and meditation can help reduce stress and foster a positive mindset. Spend a few minutes each day focusing on your breath and allowing your thoughts to come and go without judgment.

7. Challenge Negative Thoughts: When negative thoughts arise, take a moment to challenge them. Ask yourself if there's any evidence to support the thought and consider alternative perspectives.

8. Find Joy in Small Things: Look for joy and gratitude in everyday moments. Enjoy a cup of tea, listen to your favorite music, or watch a beautiful sunset.

9. Laugh and Smile: Laughter and smiles can go a long way in boosting your mood. Do something that makes you laugh, or watch a funny movie.

10. Seek Professional Support: If you're struggling to develop a positive mindset, reach out to a mental health professional. They can help you identify underlying issues and develop skills to foster a positive mindset.

Building Self-esteem and Confidence

1. Acknowledge Your Accomplishments: Celebrate the small wins and big successes you've achieved in your life. This will help you recognize that you are capable of achieving more.

2. Practice Positive Self-Talk: Speak kindly to yourself, and remind yourself of your strengths and talents.

3. Appreciate Yourself: Accept yourself and your life experiences, and be content with who you are.

4. Make Connections: Socialize with friends and family, attend community events, and stay engaged with the world.

5. Prioritize Self-Care: Take time for yourself and engage in activities that bring you joy and relaxation.

6. Pursue Hobbies and Interests: Find activities that you enjoy and can learn from.

7. Set Goals: Aim for something that excites you and challenges you.

8. Take Risks: Step outside of your comfort zone and try something new.

9. Improve Your Mindset: Focus on the positive, and find ways to be optimistic.

10. Live in the Moment: Don't worry about the past or future, and instead focus on what's happening in your life right now.

Establishing Healthy Habits and Routine

Establishing healthy habits and routines in old age is important. It can help keep the body and mind active and healthy, reduce falls and other injuries, and reduce the risk of chronic diseases such as heart disease, diabetes, and stroke. Healthy habits such as regular exercise, eating a balanced diet, and getting adequate sleep can help seniors stay physically and mentally fit and reduce the risk of developing serious health conditions. Establishing healthy habits can also help seniors stay socially connected and engaged with their community, which is important for emotional and mental well-being.

Social Support and Connection

Social support and connection play an important role in the health and well-being of older adults. Studies have consistently shown that older adults who have strong social support networks are more likely to be physically and mentally healthier, and have better cognitive functioning and quality of life.

Social support can come from family, friends, and other members of the community. It can involve emotional support, such as providing comfort and reassurance, practical support, such as helping with errands or transportation, and informational support, such as providing advice and guidance.

Connection is also important for older adults. Social connection involves engaging in activities and conversations with other people, which can help to reduce loneliness and boost mood. Activities such as hobbies, volunteering, and attending social events can all help to maintain social connections.

For those who are unable to go out, technology can provide an alternative way to stay connected.

Video-calling and messaging services such as Skype and WhatsApp can help to keep in touch with loved ones, while online forums and social media can provide an opportunity to engage with others who share similar interests or experiences.

Overall, social support and connection are essential for older adults to maintain physical, mental, and emotional well-being. There are many ways to stay connected, including in person and online, which can help to promote health and happiness in old age.

Learning New Skills and Pursuing Hobbies

1. Take Up a New Language

Learning a new language is a great way to stay mentally sharp and culturally connected in old age. Not only will it help to keep your brain active, but it can also open up a world of new opportunities and interesting conversations.

There are a variety of online, in-person, and self-study resources available to help you get started.

2. Get Creative with Art

Art is a great way to express yourself and explore new creative outlets. Whether it's painting, drawing, sculpting, or simply doodling, art can be a great way to keep your mind active and engaged. It's also a great way to express yourself and share your passions with others.

3. Try Out a New Instrument

If you've always wanted to learn an instrument, now is the time to do it! Whether it's the guitar, the piano, or the violin, learning a new instrument is a great way to stay mentally and physically active. There are a variety of online and in-person resources available to help you get started.

4. Take Up Gardening

Gardening is a great way to stay physically active and enjoy the outdoors. It's also a great way to grow your food, connect with nature, and even make a bit of extra money by selling your produce.

There are a variety of online and in-person resources available to help you get started.

5. Learn a New Craft

Whether it's crocheting, knitting, woodworking, or something else, learning a new craft is a great way to stay mentally and physically active. It's also a great way to express yourself and create something tangible. There are a variety of online and in-person resources available to help you get started.

6. Explore New Technologies

Technology is constantly changing, so it's important to stay up to date. Learning how to use new technologies can keep your mind active and open up a world of new opportunities. There are a variety of online and in-person resources available to help you get started.

CHAPTER 2

Healthy Eating and Aging

As individuals age, it is even more important to maintain a healthy diet. Eating nutritious foods can help seniors optimize their physical and mental well-being, prevent chronic diseases and improve their overall quality of life. Healthy eating in old age can benefit seniors in many ways. Eating nutrient-rich foods can help boost energy and improve overall health. Healthy eating can help seniors stay independent, maintain a healthy weight, and reduce the risk of chronic diseases such as diabetes, heart disease, and stroke. Eating a balanced diet can also help prevent osteoporosis and reduce the risk of some forms of cancer. Additionally, healthy eating can help reduce the risk of depression and improve cognitive function.

Health Benefits of Healthy Eating

1. Improved Immune System: Eating a balanced diet rich in fruits, vegetables, whole grains, and lean proteins can help boost immune system functioning, which can help seniors ward off minor illnesses and infections.

2. Reduced Risk of Heart Disease: Eating a heart-healthy diet low in saturated fat, trans fat, and cholesterol can help reduce the risk of heart disease, stroke, and other cardiovascular conditions.

3. Weight Control: Eating a nutritious and balanced diet can help seniors maintain a healthy weight, which can reduce the risk of obesity and its related health consequences.

4. Reduced Risk of Osteoporosis: Eating a healthy diet that is rich in calcium and vitamin D can help strengthen bones and reduce the risk of osteoporosis and fractures.

5. Improved Mental Health: Eating a balanced diet can help seniors stay mentally alert and cognitively sharp.

Eating nutrient-dense foods can also help improve mood and reduce the risk of developing depression.

Tips for Healthy Eating

1. Choose whole grains: Swap out white bread and white rice for whole-grain alternatives like whole-wheat bread and brown rice.

2. Eat plenty of fruits and vegetables: Fill half your plate with produce for vitamins, minerals, and fiber.

3. Choose lean proteins: Opt for lean proteins like poultry, fish, and beans.

4. Limit processed and sugary foods: Avoid processed foods, which can be high in sodium, sugar, and unhealthy fats.

6. Don't skip meals: Eating regular meals can help seniors maintain energy levels and prevent overeating.

Eating for Optimal Health

Eating for optimal health in old age involves eating a balanced and nutrient-rich diet to ensure that the body gets all the essential nutrients it needs. This includes eating plenty of fruits and vegetables, whole grains, lean proteins, dairy, and healthy fats. It is also important to limit the intake of processed and sugary foods, as well as red meat and saturated fats. Eating a balanced diet can help to reduce the risk of chronic disease, maintain muscle mass and strength, and improve overall health and well-being. Additionally, staying hydrated, getting regular physical activity, and managing stress can all help to promote optimal health as we age.

1. Eat a Balanced Diet: Eating a balanced diet is one of the most important things you can do to maintain your health as you age. Focus on a variety of nutrient-dense foods such as lean proteins, fruits, vegetables, whole grains, and healthy fats.

2. Stay Hydrated: Drinking enough water is essential for maintaining optimal health and avoiding dehydration, especially as you age. Aim for 6-8 glasses of water a day to stay properly hydrated.

3. Avoid Unhealthy Fats: Unhealthy fats, such as trans fats and saturated fats, can increase your risk for heart disease and stroke. Avoid these types of fats and opt for healthier options such as monounsaturated fats and polyunsaturated fats.

4. Get Enough Calcium and Vitamin D: As you age, your body's ability to absorb calcium and vitamin D decreases. Make sure to get enough of these essential nutrients by consuming dairy products, green leafy vegetables, and fish such as salmon or tuna.

5. Consume Less Sodium: Too much sodium can lead to high blood pressure and an increased risk of stroke. Limit your intake of canned and processed foods, which are often high in sodium.

6. Eat More Fiber: Eating enough fiber can help prevent constipation, reduce cholesterol levels, and lower your risk for heart disease. Add whole grains, fruits, and vegetables to your diet to get the most fiber.

7. Limit Alcohol and Caffeine Intake: Too much alcohol and caffeine can cause dehydration and interfere with your sleep. It's important to limit your intake of these beverages to promote healthy aging.

8. Exercise Regularly: Regular physical activity is essential for maintaining optimal health.

Nutrition and Aging

Nutrition is especially important for older adults, as nutrient needs increase and many health issues can affect the ability to get enough nutrients from food.

Protein:

Adequate protein intake is essential for maintaining muscle mass, bone health, and immune system function. A diet rich in protein-rich foods, such as lean meats, fish, dairy products, eggs, legumes, nuts, and seeds, can help meet protein needs.

Fiber:

Fiber is important for maintaining digestive health, and it can also help lower cholesterol levels and control blood sugar. Foods such as fruits, vegetables, whole grains, legumes, and nuts are good sources of fiber.

Calcium and Vitamin D:

 Low-fat dairy products, fortified cereals and juices, and dark green leafy vegetables are good sources of calcium.

Vitamin D can be obtained from fortified foods, such as milk and orange juice, as well as from exposure to sunlight.

Vitamins and Minerals:

Older adults should get enough of all the essential vitamins and minerals, including vitamins A, C, E, K, and B vitamins, as well as minerals such as iron, zinc, and magnesium. Fruits and vegetables, whole grains, legumes, nuts, and seeds are all good sources of these vitamins and minerals.

Healthy Fats:

Healthy fats, such as those found in olive oil, avocados, and nuts, can help maintain brain function and reduce the risk of heart disease.

It's also important for older adults to stay hydrated. Water is the best choice, but low-fat milk, 100% fruit juice, and other non-alcoholic beverages can also help meet fluid needs.

Healthy, Happy Aging

Finally, it's important to note that older adults should not follow fad diets, as these can be unhealthy and may not provide enough nutrients. It's important to talk to a doctor or registered dietitian to ensure that an individual's nutritional needs are being met.

Healthy Eating Plan and Aging

Changes as a result of aging can lead to health issues, such as a decrease in muscle mass, bone loss, and an increase in health problems associated with poor nutrition. Eating a healthy diet is essential for maintaining a healthy lifestyle and preventing chronic diseases. A healthy eating plan in old age should include foods that are high in protein, fiber, and essential vitamins and minerals. It should also limit unhealthy fats, added sugars, and processed foods. In this article, we will discuss the importance of creating a healthy eating plan in old age, as well as provide tips on how to create one.

Importance of a Healthy Eating Plan

Healthy, Happy Aging

A healthy eating plan is important for older adults to ensure they are getting all the essential nutrients they need. Eating a healthy diet helps to maintain muscle mass, prevent bone loss, and reduce the risk of chronic diseases such as heart disease, stroke, and diabetes. Eating a balanced diet with a variety of foods also helps to ensure that you are getting all the vitamins and minerals your body needs.

Tips for Creating a Healthy Eating Plan

1. Choose foods from all the food groups, including fruits, vegetables, grains, proteins, and dairy.

2. Limit unhealthy fats: Unhealthy fats, such as trans fats, should be limited. Foods high in trans fats include processed and fried foods. Instead, choose healthy fats such as olive oil, avocados, and nuts.

3. Choose lean proteins: Choose lean proteins such as fish, chicken, and legumes. These proteins are lower in saturated fat and higher in essential nutrients.

4. Eat foods rich in fiber: Fibrous foods such as fruits, vegetables, and whole grains are important for maintaining a healthy digestive system.

5. Limit added sugars: Eating too much-added sugar can lead to health problems such as obesity and type 2 diabetes.

6. Avoid empty calories: empty calories from sugar-sweetened drinks, processed foods, and alcohol can lead to weight gain and other health problems.

7. Drink plenty of water: Water helps to keep you hydrated and can help with digestion. Aim for 8 glasses per day, or more if you're very active.

8. Get Enough Calcium: Calcium helps to keep bones strong and can reduce the risk of osteoporosis. Good sources of calcium include dairy products and dark green leafy vegetables.

9. Watch Your Sodium Intake: Too much sodium can increase your risk of high blood pressure.

10. Get Enough Sleep: Getting enough sleep helps to keep your body functioning properly and can help reduce stress.

Creating a healthy eating plan in old age is essential for maintaining a healthy lifestyle and preventing chronic diseases. Eating a variety of foods, limiting unhealthy fats, choosing lean proteins, eating foods rich in fiber, and limiting added sugars are all important components of a healthy eating plan. Following these tips can help ensure that you are getting all the essential nutrients your body needs.

Smart Shopping and Meal Preparation

Smart shopping and meal preparation in old age can involve taking advantage of online grocery shopping and delivery services, making use of frozen meals, preparing meals in large batches, and storing them in the freezer. Many older adults may also benefit from using slow cookers, food processors, and other kitchen tools to make meal preparation easier. Additionally, using recipes that require fewer ingredients and steps can be beneficial. Finally, taking time to plan meals, create a grocery list, and purchase groceries in bulk can help older adults save time and money.

Smart shopping and meal preparation in old age can help seniors stay healthy and save money.

Healthy, Happy Aging

1. Make a shopping list: Before you hit the grocery store, make a list of the foods you need for the week. Start with the items you need for any meals you have planned, such as fruits and vegetables for a salad or ingredients for your favorite casserole. Then, fill in the rest of your list with healthy staples such as whole grains, low-fat dairy, lean proteins, and healthy fats.

2. Look for items that are on sale in larger quantities, and freeze or refrigerate what you won't use right away. This also applies to perishable items like fruits and vegetables; buy more and freeze what you won't eat right away.

3. Plan your meals: Planning your meals ahead of time can help you save time, money, and energy. Start with a few staple dishes, such as soups and casseroles, that you can make in large batches and freeze for later. Then, plan your weekly meals around those dishes. You can also plan meals around what's on sale at the store.

4. Buy frozen or canned produce: Frozen and canned fruits and vegetables are just as nutritious as fresh, and they can be more affordable. Look for items that are canned in natural juices or frozen without added sugars or sauces.

5. Use leftovers: Don't throw out leftovers! Instead, use them to create new meals. For example, use leftover chicken to make soup or use vegetables to make a stir-fry.

6. Buy pre-cut fruits and vegetables: Pre-cut fruits and vegetables can save you time and energy in the kitchen. Look for packages that are marked "ready-to-eat" or "ready-to-cook" so you know exactly what you're getting.

7. Consider food delivery services: If shopping and preparing meals is becoming too difficult, look into food delivery services. Many companies offer pre-made meals or meal kits that can be delivered right to your door.

CHAPTER 3

Dietary and Aging

As people age, their dietary needs change, and special diets may be required. Elderly individuals may benefit from diets that are low in sodium, saturated fat, and cholesterol due to their increased risk of developing certain chronic conditions. Additionally, elderly individuals may need to increase their intake of certain vitamins and minerals to help maintain their health.

To accommodate these dietary needs, it is important to focus on nutrient-dense foods that provide the most nutrition with the fewest calories. In addition to providing macronutrients, these foods contain important vitamins, minerals, and antioxidants. It is also important to limit processed and packaged foods, which are often high in sodium, saturated fat, and added sugars.

Healthy, Happy Aging

1. Protein: As people age, their protein needs remain the same, but older adults need to eat high-quality proteins that are easily digested.

2. Calcium: Older adults need at least 1,200 mg of calcium per day to maintain strong bones and ward off osteoporosis.

3. Vitamin D: Older adults should aim for 600 IU of vitamin D per day. The best sources of vitamin D are fortified dairy products, eggs, and fatty fish like salmon and tuna.

4. Fiber: Fiber is important for digestion and can help reduce the risk of heart disease, diabetes, and certain types of cancer.

5. Healthy Fats: Healthy fats, such as those found in olive oil, avocados, and nuts, can help reduce the risk of heart disease and diabetes.

6. Hydration: The elderly are at an increased risk of dehydration due to changes in their body's ability to regulate fluids. Older adults need to drink at least 8 glasses of water per day.

Understanding Food Allergies and Intolerance

Food allergies and intolerances can be difficult to manage at any age, but they can be especially challenging in old age. As we age, our immune systems become weaker and our bodies become more sensitive to food allergens. This can make it more difficult to identify and manage food allergies and intolerances.

Symptoms of food allergies and intolerances can range from mild to severe and can include hives, stomach pain, vomiting, and difficulty breathing. If left untreated, food allergies and intolerances can lead to serious health complications, including anaphylaxis, a life-threatening reaction.

The best way to manage food allergies and intolerances in old age is to be aware of the foods that may trigger a reaction. Common food allergens in older adults include milk, eggs, tree nuts, peanuts, wheat, soy, fish, and shellfish. It is also important to be aware of cross-contamination, which can occur when food allergens come into contact with other foods.

If you or a loved one has a food allergy or intolerance, it is important to talk to a doctor or allergist. They can help diagnose the allergy or intolerance and create an individualized plan to help manage the condition. This plan may include dietary changes, medications, or immunotherapy. Additionally, it is important to carry an epinephrine auto-injector at all times in case of a severe reaction.

It is also important for older adults to be aware of the signs and symptoms of food allergies and intolerances. This includes any changes in skin color, swelling of the face, lips, or tongue, difficulty breathing, and dizziness.

Finally, it is important to educate family, friends, and caregivers about food allergies and intolerances. This can help ensure that meals and snacks are prepared safely and that the individual is not exposed to allergens.

By understanding and managing food allergies and intolerances in old age, older adults can stay healthy

Eating for a Healthy Heart

Eating healthy is important at any age, but especially important as you get older. Keeping your heart healthy as you age can help you live a longer, healthier life. Here are some tips to help you eat for a healthy heart:

1. Eat a variety of nutrient-rich foods: Eating a wide variety of nutrient-rich foods from all food groups helps to keep your heart healthy. Be sure to include fruits, vegetables, whole grains, and lean proteins in your diet.

2. Limit saturated and trans fats: Eating too much saturated and trans fats can increase your risk of heart disease.

3. Eat plenty of fiber: Eating a diet high in fiber can help lower your cholesterol and reduce your risk of heart disease. Choose whole grains, fruits, and vegetables to increase your fiber intake.

4. Choose healthy fats: Eating foods that are high in healthy fats, such as omega-3 fatty acids, can help keep your heart healthy. Try to include fatty fish, walnuts, and flaxseeds in your diet.

5. Limit added sugars: Eating too much-added sugar can lead to weight gain, which can increase your risk of heart disease. Be sure to limit your intake of sugary drinks and candy.

6. Drink in moderation: Drinking too much alcohol can increase your risk of heart disease.

By following these tips, you can help keep your heart healthy as you age. Eating a balanced diet and limiting alcohol consumption will help you stay healthy and active for many years to come.

Eating for Diabetes Management

Eating for diabetes management in old age is a challenge. As we age, our metabolism slows down, making it harder to manage our blood sugar levels. Older adults may also experience loss of appetite, taste changes, difficulty preparing meals, and difficulty accessing healthy foods.

Fortunately, there are several steps you can take to help manage diabetes at an older age.

1. Eat smaller, more frequent meals. Eating several small meals throughout the day can help keep your blood sugar levels in check. Eating meals that are high in fiber and low in saturated fat can help you maintain healthy blood glucose levels.

2. Choose healthy snacks. Snacking can help prevent low blood sugar levels. Choose snacks that are nutrient-dense and low in fat, sugar, and salt.

3. Exercise regularly. Exercise is important for managing diabetes at any age.

4. Monitor your blood sugar levels. Regularly monitoring your blood sugar levels can help you identify patterns in your diabetes management and make adjustments to your diet and lifestyle.

5. Talk to your doctor. If you're having trouble managing your diabetes, make sure to talk to your doctor. They can help you develop an individualized plan to manage your diabetes and help you stay healthy.

Healthy Weight Management

As people age, it is natural for their metabolism to slow down and for them to lose some muscle mass. This can lead to weight gain, especially if their dietary and exercise habits remain unchanged. To prevent weight gain, older adults should focus on eating a balanced diet and engaging in regular physical activity. Eating smaller portion sizes and avoiding sugary and processed foods can also help. Additionally, staying socially active and engaging in hobbies can help reduce stress and improve overall mental health, which can also help with weight management.

Tips for Healthy Weight Management in Old Age

a. Eat a Balanced Diet: As you age, it is important to focus on eating a balanced diet. Avoid processed and sugary foods.

b. Exercise Regularly: Exercise can help with weight management and overall health. This can include walking, biking, swimming, dancing, or any other activity you enjoy.

c. Get Enough Sleep: Sleep is essential for maintaining a healthy weight.

d. Monitor Your Weight: Checking your weight regularly can help you stay on track with your goals.

e. Drink More Water: Drinking plenty of water can help you feel full and reduce cravings for unhealthy foods.

f. Avoid stress eating: Stress can lead to emotional eating, which can lead to weight gain. Try to find healthy ways to manage stress, such as regular exercise, meditation, or yoga.

g. Seek Support: Talking to a doctor, dietitian, or counselor can help you reach your weight management goals.

CHAPTER 4

Exercise and Aging

Exercise and physical activity are important for older adults as they can help improve overall health and wellness, reduce the risk of disease, and increase the quality of life. Exercise can help older adults maintain and improve strength, flexibility, balance, and endurance. It can also help improve mobility, decrease the risk of falls, and reduce stress, anxiety, and depression.

Physical activity is also important for older adults to maintain and improve their overall health. Research has found that regular physical activity can decrease the risk of chronic diseases such as heart disease, high blood pressure, and diabetes.

It can also reduce the risk of certain cancers and help with weight management. Physical activity can also help improve cognitive functioning and reduce feelings of depression and anxiety.

Older adults should consult with their doctor before starting a new exercise program to ensure it is appropriate for their age and health condition. It is also important to start slowly and gradually build up the intensity and duration of the activity. Low-impact activities, such as walking, swimming, or yoga, are recommended for older adults who are just starting an exercise program.

The best exercise for aging adults in old age.

As we age, it can become harder to stay active and fit. However, regular physical activity is essential for maintaining health and quality of life for aging adults. Exercise can help to reduce the risk of age-related diseases, improve physical and mental health, and enhance overall well-being.

Healthy, Happy Aging

Here are some of the best exercises for aging adults:

1. Walking: Walking is a low-impact exercise that is easy on the joints and can be done almost anywhere. It can be done indoors or outdoors and can be done as a stroll or a fast-paced power walk.

2. Swimming: Swimming is a great way to get your heart rate up while protecting your joints.

3. Water aerobics: Water aerobics is a great way for aging adults to get a good workout without putting strain on their joints.

4. Yoga: Yoga is a great exercise for all ages.

5. Tai Chi: Tai Chi is a low-impact martial art that can help to improve balance, strength, and coordination.

6. Resistance Training: Resistance training with weights or resistance bands can help improve strength and muscle mass. It is important to start slowly and use light weights or resistance bands to prevent injury.

No matter what exercise you choose, it is important to talk to your doctor before beginning any new exercise routine. Your doctor can help you determine the best exercise plan for your needs and abilities

Making the Exercise you enjoy Part of your Life

As we age, it can be difficult to maintain a regular exercise routine. The good news is that it's never too late to start. Exercise can help you stay healthy and active, and can also improve your quality of life.

The key to making exercise a part of your life at an older age is to find something that you enjoy. Whether it's swimming, biking, walking, or something else, try to find an activity that you look forward to doing.

When you find something you enjoy, make it part of your daily routine. Set aside time each day to get in some physical activity, and stick to it. Make sure to mix up the types of activities you do, so that you don't get bored.

It's also important to listen to your body. As you age, your body may not be able to handle the same vigorous exercise that it could in the past. Focus on low-impact activities, and modify exercises if necessary.

Finally, find an exercise buddy or join a class. Exercise can be more fun when you do it with others, and it can also help you stay motivated.

Making exercise a part of your life at an older age is not only beneficial for your physical health, but also for your mental health.

CHAPTER 5

Sleeping and Aging

Aging is a natural process of life, and it brings with it both physical and emotional changes. As we age, our bodies become more vulnerable to age-related diseases and conditions, and we may experience physical and mental declines. Sleep is an essential part of the aging process and can be a key factor in maintaining physical and mental health during the later years of life.

The effects of aging on sleep can vary from person to person, but the most common are shorter and less restful sleep, decreased alertness during the day, and an increased risk for insomnia. An older adult may also find it more difficult to fall asleep and stay asleep and may experience more frequent waking episodes during the night. In addition, older adults are more likely to suffer from daytime sleepiness, which can impair their ability to function while awake.

There are several steps older adults can take to ensure they are getting the restful sleep they need. Establishing a regular sleep schedule and avoiding caffeine and alcohol before bedtime can help to promote better sleep. Additionally, engaging in regular exercise and avoiding naps during the day can help to improve sleep quality. For those who suffer from insomnia or other sleep disorders, seeking medical help may be necessary to ensure they are getting the rest they need.

Aging and sleep are intertwined, and understanding the effects of aging on sleep can help to ensure older adults are getting the restful sleep they need to stay healthy. With the right lifestyle changes, older adults can maintain good sleep quality and enjoy the many benefits that come with a well-rested life.

Tips for Better Sleep

• Establish a regular sleep schedule

• Make sure your bedroom is conducive to sleep.

• Avoid caffeine and alcohol in the evening.

• Exercise regularly, but not too close to bedtime.

• Avoid looking at screens at least one hour before bed.

• Try relaxation techniques, such as yoga, meditation, or progressive muscle relaxation.

• Talk to your doctor about any medications or supplements that might be disrupting your sleep.

Common Age-related Sleep Issues

1. Difficulty Falling Asleep

- Causes: Stress, caffeine consumption, irregular sleep schedule, poor sleep habits

- Solutions: Avoid caffeine consumption close to bedtime, establish a regular sleep schedule, practice relaxation techniques such as deep breathing, meditation, and progressive muscle relaxation, and create a comfortable sleep environment

2. Difficulty Staying Asleep

- Causes: Stress, anxiety, pain, sleep apnea, restless leg syndrome

- Solutions: Reduce stress and anxiety with relaxation techniques, practice good sleep hygiene, consider using a white noise machine, and talk to your doctor if you experience chronic pain.

3. Early Morning Waking

- Causes: Anxiety, stress, medical conditions, shift work

- Solutions: Establish a regular sleep schedule, practice relaxation techniques, create a comfortable sleep environment, and talk to your doctor if you suspect a medical condition or if you work shifts

How to improve Sleep as you Age

1. Avoid Caffeine: Caffeine is a stimulant that can interfere with sleep, so as you age, it's important to

minimize your intake. Avoid consuming caffeine late in the day, as it can interfere with your ability to fall asleep and stay asleep.

2. Exercise Regularly: Regular exercise can help you get better sleep as you age. Exercise can help your body regulate its circadian rhythm, which is the body's internal clock that helps regulate sleep patterns.

3. Stick to a Sleep Schedule: As you age, it can be difficult to keep a consistent sleep schedule. Try to maintain a schedule of going to bed and waking up at the same time each day, even on weekends. This will help your body adjust to a consistent sleep pattern.

4. Reduce Stress: Stress can interfere with sleep, so it's important to find ways to reduce stress as you age. Try exercising, practicing mindfulness and meditation, or talking to a friend or family member.

5. Create a Comfortable Environment: Make sure your bedroom is comfortable and quiet. Make sure the temperature is comfortable and that the lighting is dim.

Also, avoid using electronics near bedtime, as the light from screens can interfere with sleep.

Healthy Sleep Routine

1. Establish a regular sleep schedule: Establishing a regular sleep schedule is important for maintaining healthy sleep habits.

An aged person should aim to go to bed and wake up at the same time each day. This will help the body adjust to a consistent sleep pattern.

2. Regular physical activity can help reduce stress and anxiety, improve sleep quality, and reduce the risk of health problems.

3. Avoid stimulants before bed: Caffeine, nicotine, and alcohol can all interfere with sleep. Aged persons should avoid caffeine and nicotine close to bedtime. If alcohol is consumed, it should be done in moderation and at least two hours before bedtime.

4. Create a comfortable sleep environment: A comfortable sleep environment can help promote better rest. Choose a mattress and pillow that are comfortable and supportive, and keep the bedroom cool and dark.

5. Relax before bed: A relaxing pre-bed routine can help reduce stress and anxiety and prepare the body for sleep. Aged persons can try activities such as reading, listening to calming music, or taking a warm bath.

6. Limit screen time before bed: The blue light from screens can interfere with sleep. Aged persons should avoid using screens close to bedtime and should instead focus on calming activities.

7. Avoid napping during the day: Daytime napping can interfere with nighttime sleep. Aged persons should avoid taking long naps during the day and should instead focus on getting enough sleep at night.

Natural sleep Aids and Supplements

1. Chamomile Tea: Chamomile tea is a popular herbal remedy for insomnia. It contains compounds that may help relax the body and mind, making it easier to fall asleep.

2. Melatonin: Melatonin is a hormone naturally produced by the body that helps regulate sleep. Taking a melatonin supplement can help improve sleep quality and reduce insomnia in seniors.

3. Valerian Root: Valerian root is an herb that has been used for centuries to treat insomnia. It contains compounds that may help reduce anxiety and improve sleep quality.

4. Lavender Oil: Lavender oil is a popular natural remedy for sleep problems. Its calming and soothing properties can help reduce anxiety and improve sleep quality.

5. Magnesium: Magnesium is an important mineral that can help improve sleep quality. It can help relax the body, reduce anxiety, and promote deeper sleep.

6. B Vitamins: B vitamins are important for overall health, but they can also help improve sleep quality. B vitamins can help regulate hormones, reduce stress, and promote relaxation.

Alternative and Complementary Therapies for Sleep Disorder

1. Yoga: Yoga is effective in improving sleep quality in older adults. Yoga includes stretching, breathing, and relaxation exercises that can help reduce stress and improve relaxation, which can help improve sleep quality.

2. Meditation: Meditation is a mind-body practice that can help improve mental and physical well-being.

Research has found that meditation can help improve sleep quality in older adults, as it can help reduce stress and anxiety, which can be beneficial to sleep.

3. Aromatherapy: Aromatherapy is the use of essential oils to promote health and well-being. Aromatherapy is effective in improving sleep quality in older adults, as it can help reduce stress and anxiety, which can be beneficial to sleep.

4. Acupuncture: Acupuncture is an ancient Chinese practice that involves inserting thin needles into specific points on the body. Research has found that acupuncture can help improve sleep quality in older adults, as it can help reduce stress and anxiety, which can be beneficial to sleep.

5. Herbal Remedies: Herbal remedies are natural treatments based on plants and herbs. Herbal remedies are effective in improving sleep quality in older adults, as they can help reduce stress and anxiety, which can be beneficial to sleep.

Benefits of Supplements for Anti-aging

1. Antioxidants: Antioxidants are compounds found in foods that are believed to help protect the body from damage caused by free radicals. Free radicals are molecules that can cause oxidative stress, which is linked to aging and diseases like cancer and heart disease. Some of the most potent antioxidants include vitamins C and E, carotenoids, and polyphenols.

2. Collagen: Collagen is a type of protein that is essential for the structure of the skin and other connective tissues. Taking collagen supplements can help replenish the body's supply of this important protein, helping to keep skin looking firmer and smoother.

3. Omega-3 Fatty Acids: Omega-3 fatty acids are essential fatty acids that have been linked to several health benefits, including anti-aging. Omega-3s can help reduce inflammation, which is believed to play a

role in aging. They can also help keep skin hydrated and protect against sun damage.

4. Coenzyme Q10: Coenzyme Q10 (CoQ10) is a compound that is naturally produced by the body. It plays an important role in energy production and is believed to help protect against cell damage caused by free radicals. CoQ10 supplements can help replenish the body's levels of this important compound and may have anti-aging benefits.

5. Resveratrol: Resveratrol is a compound found in red wine and certain plants. It has been linked to anti-aging effects, as it's believed to help protect against oxidative stress.

Taking resveratrol supplements can help increase the body's levels of this important compound and may help protect against the signs of aging.

CHAPTER 6

Mental Health and Anti-aging

Healthy, Happy Aging

Mental health and anti-aging are closely related concepts. Mental health is the overall state of emotional, psychological, and physical well-being. Individuals need to maintain good mental health to age well. Anti-aging refers to strategies and techniques used to slow down or reverse the biological aging process. Research has shown that a healthy lifestyle, including mental health, can help to slow down the aging process.

Maintaining good mental health helps support the body's immune system and can reduce the risk of age-related diseases. Stress management, exercise, adequate sleep, and a balanced diet are all important for maintaining a healthy lifestyle and keeping the body and mind healthy.

Additionally, positive relationships, hobbies, and activities that promote emotional well-being are important for maintaining mental health.

In addition to the lifestyle changes mentioned above, some treatments and therapies can help improve mental health. Cognitive behavioral therapy, psychotherapy, and meditation can help individuals cope better with daily stressors and reduce the risk of age-related diseases. Anti-aging treatments and products may also be used to reduce the visible signs of aging. These may include topical creams, lasers, and injectables.

Overall, mental health and anti-aging are closely related concepts, and it is important to maintain good mental health to age well. A healthy lifestyle, including stress management, exercise, adequate sleep, and a balanced diet, can support the body's immune system and help to slow down the aging process. Additionally, treatments and therapies can help improve mental health, while anti-aging treatments and products can reduce the visible signs of aging.

Mental Health Strategies for Anti-Aging

1. Make Exercise a Priority: Exercise is one of the best things you can do to help keep your body and mind healthy as you age. Incorporating regular physical activity into your life can help reduce stress, improve your mood, and boost your energy levels.

2. Eat a Healthy Diet: Eating a balanced diet rich in fruits, vegetables, whole grains, and lean proteins is essential for optimal health as you age. Avoid processed foods and sugary drinks, and focus on getting essential vitamins and minerals to keep your body functioning at its best.

3. Get Enough Sleep: Adequate sleep is essential for both physical and mental health. Aim to get 7-8 hours of sleep each night to help stay energized throughout the day and reduce stress.

4. Stay Socially Connected: Isolation can harm mental health, so it's important to stay socially connected as you age. Reach out to friends and family, join a club or volunteer organization, or take a class to meet new people and keep your mind active.

5. Practice Relaxation Techniques: Relaxation techniques such as yoga, meditation, and deep breathing can help reduce stress and improve mental health. Incorporate these activities into your daily routine to help keep your mind and body balanced

6. Manage Stress: Stress can take a toll on your physical and mental health, so it's important to find ways to

manage stress levels. Exercise, relaxation techniques, and spending time with loved ones can all help reduce stress and promote mental health.

7. Seek Professional Help: If you're feeling overwhelmed or having difficulty managing your mental health, don't hesitate to seek professional help. A mental health professional can help you develop coping strategies and provide support as you age.

Stress Management

Stress has been linked to accelerated aging in several ways. Psychological stress can cause the body to produce higher levels of the hormone cortisol, which is known to suppress the immune system, making the body less capable of fighting off infections and illnesses. This can lead to an increased risk of developing chronic conditions and diseases, as well as a shorter lifespan. Additionally, chronic psychological stress has been linked to changes in cellular structures, leading to premature aging in the form of wrinkles, gray hair, and other signs of aging. Finally, psychological stress can lead to unhealthy behaviors such as smoking or drinking, which can further damage the body and speed up the aging process

The Effect of Stress on Aging.

Stress is an inevitable part of life, but it can have a significant impact on the aging process. Research has shown that chronic stress can increase the risk of developing age-related diseases, such as dementia and Alzheimer's, as well as reduce lifespan.

Stress accelerates the aging process in several ways. It can suppress the immune system, making the body more vulnerable to illnesses and infections.

It can also raise the body's levels of the hormone cortisol, which is linked with inflammation and cell damage. In addition, stress can cause changes in the body's metabolism, leading to an accelerated breakdown of cells and an increased risk of age-related diseases.

Stress can also cause changes in behavior and emotions, such as increased irritability, depression, and anxiety. These changes can lead to a decrease in physical activity, poor sleep habits, and unhealthy eating habits, which can all contribute to accelerated aging.

To minimize the effects of stress on the aging process, it is important to take steps to reduce stress levels. This can include engaging in regular physical activity, getting enough sleep, eating a healthy diet, and engaging in activities that promote relaxation and well-being. It is also important to seek help from a mental health professional if stress is becoming unmanageable.

Stress Management Strategies

Stress management strategies can help people take control of their stress and reduce its harmful effects on their daily lives. Here are some strategies that can be used to manage stress:

1. Regular exercise can help reduce stress levels and the risk of developing physical and mental health problems.

2. Relaxation Techniques: Relaxation techniques such as deep breathing, progressive muscle relaxation, and guided imagery can help reduce stress and improve overall health.

3. Cognitive Behavioral Therapy (CBT): CBT is a form of psychotherapy that helps people identify and change negative thinking patterns and behaviors that can lead to stress.

4. Time Management: Proper time management can help reduce stress levels by ensuring that tasks are

completed on time and that adequate time is set aside for relaxation.

5. Healthy Diet: Eating a healthy diet can help reduce stress levels and improve overall health.

6. Social Support: Having a strong social support system can help reduce stress levels by providing emotional support and understanding.

7. Meditation: Meditation is a form of mental exercise that can help reduce stress and improve overall health.

8. Sleep: Getting an adequate amount of sleep can help reduce stress levels and improve overall health.

9. Mindfulness: Mindfulness is a form of meditation that focuses on being aware of the present moment and accepting it without judgment.

10. Positive Self-Talk: Positive self-talk can help reduce stress by replacing negative thoughts with more positive ones.

CHAPTER 7

Skincare and Anti-aging

The best way to combat the signs of aging is to develop a good skincare routine that is tailored to your skin type. This should include cleansers, moisturizers, sunscreen, and, depending on your needs, products such as serums, retinoids, and exfoliants.

Cleansers, such as gentle soaps or mild foaming cleansers, help remove dirt, oil, and impurities from the skin.

Moisturizers are essential for keeping the skin hydrated. Look for products that contain ingredients such as hyaluronic acid that help lock in moisture for a more youthful complexion.

Healthy, Happy Aging

Sunscreen is important for protecting the skin from sun damage, which can cause premature aging. A broad-spectrum sunscreen with SPF 30 or higher should be applied every day, even on cloudy days.

Serums are lightweight products that can help target specific skin concerns, such as uneven skin tone or fine lines. Look for ones that contain antioxidants and peptides.

Retinoids are a form of vitamin A that can help reduce the appearance of wrinkles, boost collagen production, and even out skin tone.

Exfoliants help remove dead skin cells and promote cell turnover for a brighter, smoother complexion.

With a regular skincare routine that focuses on cleansing, moisturizing, protecting, and treating, you can help reduce the signs of aging and keep your skin looking young and healthy.

Major Benefits of Skin Care

1. Reduced appearance of wrinkles and fine lines: Skincare can help reduce the appearance of wrinkles and fine lines that develop with age due to sun exposure and the loss of collagen and elastin in the skin. Regular moisturizing, exfoliating, and using products that contain anti-aging ingredients like retinol can help reduce the appearance of wrinkles and keep skin looking youthful.

2. Improved skin tone: Skincare helps to improve skin tone by boosting collagen production, which helps to even out discoloration and other signs of aging. Using products with antioxidants, such as vitamin C and green tea extract, helps to protect the skin from environmental damage and improve the skin's overall tone.

3. Reduced dryness: As we age, our skin naturally becomes drier and thinner, so it's important to use products that help to hydrate and protect the skin. Moisturizers, hydrating masks, and serums are great for locking in moisture and reducing dryness.

4. Reduced puffiness and bags: Skincare can help reduce puffiness and bags under the eyes. Using products that contain caffeine and hyaluronic acid can help to reduce puffiness, while products with antioxidants can help to protect the delicate skin around the eyes.

5. Improved skin elasticity: Skincare helps to improve skin elasticity by boosting collagen production and protecting against environmental damage. Using products with retinol can help stimulate collagen production, while products with antioxidants can help protect the skin from environmental damage.

6. Reduced sagging: Skincare can help reduce sagging by improving skin elasticity. Using products with retinol and antioxidants can help stimulate collagen production and protect the skin from environmental damage.

7. Improved skin texture: Skincare can help to improve skin texture by exfoliating,

which helps to remove dead skin cells and reduce the appearance of dullness. Products such as masks and scrubs can help to improve skin texture and give skin a more youthful appearance.

8. Reduced age spots: Skincare can help reduce age spots by using products with anti-aging ingredients like retinol and antioxidants. These ingredients help to reduce the appearance of age spots and protect the skin from further damage.

9. Reduced hyperpigmentation: Skincare can help to reduce hyperpigmentation, which is a common sign of aging. Products with vitamin C and niacinamide can help to lighten dark spots and even out skin tone.

10. Improved overall skin health: Skincare can help to improve overall skin health by providing the skin with the nutrients it needs, protecting it from environmental damage, and reducing signs of aging. Using a combination of moisturizers, exfoliants, and serums can help to keep skin healthy and looking its best.

Skincare Routines

1. Cleanser: Old people should use a gentle cleanser that is specifically designed for aging skin. Look for cleansers that have moisturizing and nourishing ingredients, such as hyaluronic acid, jojoba oil, or aloe vera. Avoid cleansers that contain harsh or abrasive ingredients, as these can irritate the skin.

2. Toner: A toner helps to remove any residue left on the skin after cleansing, as well as helps to balance the skin's pH level. Opt for a toner that is alcohol-free and contains soothing ingredients, such as chamomile or green tea.

3. Moisturizer: Aging skin needs extra hydration and moisturizers specifically formulated for mature skin are ideal. Look for a moisturizer that contains antioxidants and anti-aging ingredients, such as retinol, peptides, and hyaluronic acid.

4. Eye Cream: The skin around the eyes is especially delicate and prone to dryness, so it's important to use a specialized eye cream.

Look for an eye cream that contains ingredients such as caffeine, peptides, and niacinamide, which can help to reduce puffiness and dark circles.

5. Sunscreen: Sunscreen is a must for every age group, but it's especially important for older people who have thinner skin.

6. Facial Oil: Facial oils are great for adding extra hydration and nourishment to aging skin. Look for facial oils that contain natural oils, such as argan oil, jojoba oil, and rosehip oil.

 7. Exfoliate: Using a gentle exfoliant once or twice a week will help to remove dead skin cells, leaving the skin feeling soft and smooth.

8. Treat: Using a serum or cream that contains ingredients like hyaluronic acid, vitamin C, and retinol can help to reduce the appearance of wrinkles, age spots, and other signs of aging.

9. Mask: Using a hydrating, soothing mask a few times a week can help to provide the skin with an extra boost of moisture and nutrients.

Conclusion

To age healthily and happily, one must remain physically active and engaged in meaningful activities, maintain a healthy diet, stay socially connected, and take steps to safeguard their mental health. The book also emphasizes the importance of having a positive attitude and outlook as we age, which can help us accept and embrace the changes that come with aging. Finally, the book encourages us to take charge of our aging process and to make the most of the years ahead.

www.ingramcontent.com/pod-product-compliance
Lightning Source LLC
Chambersburg PA
CBHW051655250726
48653CB00007B/2683